Parkinson's Disease

Looking Down the Barrel

Parkinson's Disease

Looking Down the Barrel

A Deputy Sheriff's Midlife Memoirs

Richard Secklin

Nettfit Publishing

Contact: Richard Secklin

Nettfit Publishing

3404 S 20th Street

Milwaukee, WI 53215

About the Author

Richard Secklin is a Cum Laude graduate from Lubbock
Christian University with a Bachelor of Science in
Organizational Management. Richard was a career law
enforcement officer in Texas and an instructor for the
Texas Commission on Law Enforcement Officer Standards
and Education. Richard held the highest attainable Master
Peace Officer License in Texas. Richard was diagnosed with
Parkinson's disease in 2003.

Prelude

I am four years into my diagnosis and living with Parkinson's disease (PD). My hand is shaking, not because of Parkinson's but because I'm looking down the barrel of a gun. My finger is on the trigger. The room is spinning.

My wife had dissolved our 18 year marriage and I blamed the Parkinson's. My son could no longer handle living with me and he had decided to move away too.

I'm about to vomit. My finger twitches.

I was no longer a cop: I had quit my job without notice. They never knew I had tried marijuana to relieve my PD symptoms while working for the department, and the guilt I felt was overwhelming.

I can't catch my breath.

I will not get into Heaven if I do this. It doesn't matter. I hate God. *I am on the precipice of death.*

*****

This is a story of my midlife encounter of getting diagnosed and living with Parkinson's disease. Like all PD'ers, we struggle through our own physical and/or psychological disasters and triumphs. These are my personal experiences with depression, confusion, the hate for God, and the on-going transition of this diagnosis, including my symptoms, connecting with support groups, attaining proper medical testing and treatment and finally, the survival of living with PD.

I dedicate this book to my youngest son: an unintentional liberator of my idiosyncratic sickness. Unbeknown to him at *that* moment in time - he saved me from myself.

*****

Most likely you will find yourself sitting in a doctor's office surrounded by charts and pictures on the walls. These pictures depict the brain and spine. It is a Neurology doctor you're seeing because of a myriad of symptoms that you have been dealing with.

A nurse comes out and calls a name. It's not yours. You observe a women stand up but you are confused because a man's name had been called. The woman turns and helps the man sitting next to her stand up. He has trouble. Once standing, it appears that he intends to start walking to the waiting nurse who patiently holds the door open. His leg starts shaking. His brain is telling his leg to pick up and move but his leg has trouble responding. He seems to be hesitating. All of a sudden, as if someone pushed him from behind, he almost runs across the room - but only for a few steps, and then he finally gains control and he slows down. Your fear starts to take hold. You take a deep breath. *Your* name will be called soon.

****

Looking Down the Barrel

I am hysterically crying as I look down the barrel of my Glock 17. I am thinking, my temple or in my mouth?

I had looked down the barrel of my gun many times before but not like this. It was never loaded when I cleaned it. This time it *was* loaded, with a special hollow point bullet authorized for police officers only. I knew my gun would not misfire. I had been a career law enforcement officer, a supervisor, an instructor and a previous SWAT team member. Life could not have been better before being diagnosed with Parkinson's disease. But, from time to time, life throws something at us. And every once and awhile it's something really big. I was not ready for *this*.

I am sitting at the edge of my bed sweating. My hand is shaking; my finger twitching- on the trigger. My life flashes before me.

I had survived psychological and physical events before. I had endured infidelity and divorce. I had survived a broken neck, and had my chest opened up for the removal of a large cyst.

But now I am losing everything. I have Parkinson's disease and my symptoms are steadily advancing.

I was a Christian but lost my faith in God, and now I had lost all hope.

I am quitting life. I am giving up. The gun feels heavy in my hand.

And then I heard a noise. It was the front door closing as my son arrives home from school. I didn't even realize what time it was.

Do we ever know what time it is the moment we die?

I slid the gun under my pillow and wiped the tears from my face. My sixteen year old son walked into my bedroom to let me know he was home. I tried to maintain my composure.

"Are you ok, dad?" He could tell I had been crying. I lied when I told him I'd be alright. But, he was a smart young man: an honor student, and aware that, often, due to my Parkinson's disease, I would get discouraged. He also knew I had been very depressed over my recent divorce from his mother. He had been depressed himself, as his mother left both of us.

I was a great father and a good husband - at least that's what she told me when she confessed she was in love with someone else.

Why then?

I never ran around, never cheated. I was always home. I was a good provider, and a coach on my son's football team.

Was it because I had Parkinson's?

I was engulfed in my own loss, my own disease, and not even thinking about what my son was going through. He had lost his mother too- in a sense - she was living in another state. His father has Parkinson's and just gave up

his career in law enforcement-which didn't make any sense

at all.

My moods were all over the place, and I had become

intolerable to live with. Even though he could have

graduated at the age of sixteen, and he knew that moving to

another state would mean yet another year of school -

because of me, my son had decided to do exactly that. Not

that he really *wanted* to move away from his friends; no

sixteen year old does. But, because I seemed to be going off

the deep end, engulfed in my own remorse: that was his

decision. Do all diseases cause this much turmoil in

families?

My son is unaware of the gun under my pillow.

****

Mad at God

My wife and I had been attending church regularly.

We held Bible study classes every Friday in our living room and had done so for the last three years. In my thirties I was baptized as a Methodist Christian and ministered the word of God every chance I had. I was employed as a detention deputy and a supervisor working in the sheriff's office which gave me a chance to talk or "minister" with inmates from time to time. Imagine how great it felt when ex-inmates approached you on the street to thank you for treating them with respect while they were incarcerated and speaking the Word. Law Enforcement can be a thankless job unless one tries to make a difference.

None of that matters anymore. I have Parkinson's and now I am the one that needs ministering. Is God testing me?

* * * * *

I wondered why God would do this to *me. Why did I get Parkinson's?* Did I get the disease from the years working above the ship's propellers when I was enlisted in the Navy?

Maybe - I remember breathing diesel fuel all day. To another extreme, maybe I got this disease because of my hereditary genes. Through my Jewish heritage I can be classified as an Ashkenazi Jew with ancestry from Lithuania - Russia. Ashkenazi Jews are more likely to acquire Parkinson's disease if they carry the G2019S DNA mutation: an important cause of both familial and sporadic Parkinson's disease. I discovered these facts through research. (My research is ongoing)

God only knows how I got this chronic progressive disease. Whatever, I was still mad at God and blaming Him. I was expecting an email from Him anytime that reads:

You should not have kicked the cat!

LOL from God DO NOT REPLY TO THIS MESSAGE.

****

Depression

Was it my Parkinson's disease or my depression that chased

my wife away? My wife was a registered nurse; she certainly

knew the outcome of Parkinson's disease.

Whatever happened to the marriage vows "in sickness and health?"

Depression is only one part of Parkinson's disease and

she knew I was dealing with that. I sure felt it too.

Uncomfortably adjusting myself in my bed with the gun still hidden

under my pillow, my son tells me he loves me.

I suddenly realize I could never pull the trigger and

make life even worse for him than it already was.

What the hell was I thinking?

He was already struggling with the divorce and loss of

his mother. She had left the two of us and moved out of

state with her boyfriend.

"Everything will be ok, I love you dad" he said.

I told him, "I love you too son."

He told me that maybe I should move back to

Milwaukee. I had other children living there that needed me

too. My other two children from a previous marriage

included three grandchildren as well.

What a strong intelligent young man he was at only

sixteen years old. He knew I needed family. Even in his own

life's blameless changing circumstances, he was thinking

about what was best for me.

I lay crying after he left my room; still depressed and still mad at God.

But, what I almost did would have been unforgivable,

and I now realized that I needed to remain strong for him,

for everyone.

****

My PD Diagnosis

I began having PD symptoms during college in 2002.

"Hey dad" my son said while we sat at the coffee table, "try this beat." We were sitting in our living room watching television and he was attempting to tap a beat on the table. Remembering a beat I used to play on the bongo drums when I was his age I countered with different beat.

"No try this one," I said, as I haphazardly taped away.

Attempting to drum out a familiar beat did not produce the outcome I had expected. Thinking for a second I had forgotten the rhythm I tried it again. Something was happening with my right hand and I sat there bewildered and stared at it. My hand appeared to be having spasms but every once in awhile my hand obeyed my brain. Still staring, I opened and closed my hand and I noticed my fingers were quivering. I think my heart stopped for a moment. I walked into the other room and showed my wife. I cannot recall what was discussed but one thing we knew for sure was that I needed to make an appointment with my doctor.

I was almost finished with my degree program when I first noticed the dexterity problems. After the first visit with my general practitioner, he scheduled a number of tests and referred me to a neurologist.

I showed my hand quivers to a fellow student as we drove to campus. I had already been thinking that my problem could be either Multiple Sclerosis or Parkinson's and I remember talking to him about the irony of being diagnosed with something just as I'm-finishing college! The foresight and cognitive combination of *what if* and *student loans* did not even enter my mind.

*****

I was diagnosed with Parkinson's disease in 2003. My diagnosis came four years before I found myself looking down the barrel of my gun. I was working in Midland Texas. I was a deputy sheriff and a supervisor while attending Lubbock Christian University as an adult learner in college. I worked full-time, coached football every night, and attended games on weekends. My degree program was an eighteen month program requiring 48 credit hours. I needed an additional 26 credit hours of supporting classes. It was my goal to finally get my Bachelor's degree before I reached fifty. I completed 74 credits in an eighteen month period attending school, work, and coaching football. In addition I somehow managed to attain the top award for my research project. Glancing back, *if I only had this energy today!*

*****

Before moving to Texas, I had worked at various industrial plants in Milwaukee years earlier. I mention this because Parkinson's disease might be caused from environmental hazards we work in. As a cabinet maker for six years, I worked in spray booths for the lamination process in countertops. I worked as a machine fabricator welding for three years. I also owned my own health club, but one could ask what chemical or environmental hazards are around a gym? Well, I was a competitive national bodybuilder and yes, I sometimes used steroids.

This is something all of us do when confronted with a disease. We try to figure out where our actions or choices in life might have made a difference. Would I have Parkinson's if I had not worked as a cabinet maker? Did steroids cause this? What if I would not have moved out of state? Maybe it's all those oil wells in Texas. If it's because of kicking the cat, I most likely would have kicked the cat one or twice wherever I lived! "WTF" - emailed to God was returned as - "no reply@domain"

I had lived in New Mexico for nine years where I operated and owned the gym and worked at a few prisons. Later I moved to Midland Texas and continued my career working in Law Enforcement. I advanced to the fourth highest peace office license any cop in Texas could achieve:

a Master Peace Officer. I then attained a licensed as a law enforcement instructor for the Texas Commission on Law Enforcement Standards and Education (TCLEOSE). I had worked as a SWAT team member, as a jail supervisor, and as a computer administrator for the department. I attained an Associate of Applied Science degree in Criminal Justice and later attained my Bachelor of Science in Organizational Management. I succeeded and graduated Cum Laude from Lubbock Christian University (LCU). Awarded in my community, I received "Officer of the Year" and was honored by the Midland Crime Prevention Commission.

Before Parkinson's some around the shop (Sheriff's Office) called me the *golden boy*. I was a jack of all trades. Now in retrospect, I wonder if the stress of it all could have initially caused my Parkinson's disease symptoms. I keep trying to find a reason.

My right hand would freeze up and my dexterity was diminishing. I thought Carpel Tunnel - probably from all the research papers I wrote. I wish!

I continued my research and medical examinations to find out what was happening with my right side of my body. "What happened to your foot?" someone would ask when they observed my difficulty in walking. "Why is it that when you walk you don't swing your right arm?"

I was a Sergeant - still wearing a uniform when my first PD symptoms developed. I recall that my right arm would not swing while walking and my hand would freeze- fingers tight, palm cupped open. Looking in the mirror my reflection was at the ready draw. *It fricklin looked like I was getting ready to draw my gun!* I thought of actor Richard Boon portrayed as a gunslinger in the 1957 television series "Have Gun will Travel" but at this moment it was me, Richard - *Half Man will Travel.*

****

Parkinson's is a disease that affects one's ability to move. It is an incurable progressive disease that many times starts out affecting one side of the body (unilateral) and later sometimes develops into (bilateral) complications affecting both sides. Young onset PD is when people under 40 years in age get this disease like Michael J. Fox. I was fifty when I started having problems but this was still too young for me! Many older people get the disease as the brain loses dopamine production.

Parkinson's disease can cause muscle rigidity, problems with one's gait, tremors, and even changes in speech. It can cause depression, cognitive problems, sleep disturbances, panic attacks, anxiety or problems with swallowing. It affects us all differently. Even the progression is different as some people diagnosed in the year I was are worse off than me. I am writing this story in 2010 - eight years into my diagnosis and my symptoms are still unilateral. With the exception of my new diagnosis of bipolar problems I am doing ok.

No I'm not - yes I am! No I'm not! — Whatever!

*****

Throughout the first few years of PD onset, doctors have to juggle different medications to see what works best. During this time I was having trouble sleeping and averaging three hours a night. With the minor PD symptoms I was still able to finish my college degree and work day shift of 40 hours per week. Sleeping so few hours per night gave me more time to work on my computer repair hobby. This hobby grew out of the garage and I then decided to build a big shop in my back yard. I enjoyed buying old PC's that I acquired from various auctions and repaired and resold them. It was a great hobby and I was very busy. I licensed my hobby as a business and called it *"Rebootyourpc.com."*

When I licensed the business I classified it as a *not for profit business* since I gave many of the computers away to people in need. Unfortunately, the city listed it as *Now for Profit*. It did not matter; my Parkinson's disease was starting to interfere with everything anyway.

Give a man a shop and he's in heaven! Give a man Parkinson's and he's not half the man he used to be! - Rebootme God.

I found that even my few hours of sleep were restless ones. I didn't know if it was because of the disease or the medicine but I would find myself tossing and turning every night. I felt that my mind would not rest so I would get out of bed and go in the shop and tinker with the computers all night.

When doctors prescribe PD medications they may not know the right dosage or combination to give. My brain needed dopamine but what happens if my brain gets too much? I think the beginning management of my medication caused my brain to become hyperactive. I found myself cleaning, working in the yard, tinkering, doing anything to stay busy. My sleepless nights most certainly had an effect on my anxiety and depression as it became a vicious cycle feeding upon itself resulting in panic attacks, cognitive problems and confusion. I call this a Parkinson's *SHARK* attack;

Sleepless – **H**yperactive - **A**nxiety - **R**eproduced – **K**ook – **ATTACK**.

After working in the shop all night, and then watching the sun come up, I would take a shower and go to work at the Sheriff's Office. That interfered with my alertness at work. If my physical ailments did not cripple me, my mental vigilance was diminished from lack of sleep. That's quite worrisome when working in a detention facility. I remember once taking a 10 minute nap in the captain's office when he was out, with the lieutenant's permission of course. These naps are essential for People with Parkinson's (PwPs).

I was also hit with a few cognitive problems when it came to compiling reports, a function I performed on a daily basis. I would find myself staring at the monitor screen trying to figure out a procedure as I tried to understand what I was doing wrong when a report would not provide the results I needed. This was a program in Microsoft Access that I had built! Talk about frustration! I realized that when I rested for a few minutes, my mental faculties would return to normal. It's so amazing how a ten minute nap helps. I recommend that if you feel you need one, take one.

Now I lay me down to nap,

To get a dopamine zap.

But if I wake before mind sync,

I'll need a shrink I think.

My Parkinson symptoms affected the right side of my body and progressively my right hand's dexterity started to diminish.

What the hell!

I just had this shop built, and I just finished college. What's going to happen to me? How fast is this disease going to progress? What was going through my mind was that I just finished college ($15,000 in student loans), I just spent six grand on a shop in my back yard, and now I was having problems using my right hand that interfered with many things. Lucky for me at that time I did not know my wife was going to leave us. But as Christians we should always be thankful.

No, to hell with God! I was still mad at Him. Maybe He is a *She* because a He God wouldn't do this to a fellow man. It's got to be a test of faith or did I kick the dog once too?

OK then - *Thank God I'm left handed.*

If all of this wasn't bad enough, politics at work were boiling over. County commissioners may have pressured the sheriff to make an administrative adjustment in the detention facility. I was a sergeant but also the assistant administrator for our UNIX law enforcement software program we used. When the captain in the detention facility unexpectedly retired after thirty years with the S.O., they had to use *me* to take up some of the slack for new software installation. I wanted to remain in the detention facility as it was my wish to become an administrator. *That's* why I attained my B.S. degree in Management. The sheriff transferred me out of the detention facility to work on computers; but my right hand does not agree.

Oh I see! Now I have to use my right hand even more.

Go figure! *Really*, God?

*****

Compassion

I recall a local Neurologist performing a spinal tap in his office checking for neurological system disorders. For a spinal tap (lumbar puncture), a sample of cerebrospinal fluid is withdrawn with a needle and sent to a laboratory for examination. The doctor had an office in Odessa Texas but had just opened this new office in Midland. In fact, I think I might have been his first patient in the Midland office that morning. He had no nurses on staff at the time and it was his receptionist's first day. She assisted him in his attempt to retrieve spinal fluid from my lumbar area. Well, who else would help him? They were the only two people there besides me, the reluctant patient! On the doctor's unsuccessful fourth attempt to retrieve spinal fluid from by back, I yelled at him and said, "Enough!"

Now I understand a spinal tap is an evasive outpatient procedure and performed in many clinics but being prepared is also having the right people on staff to assist. I was a patient that was in fear that I had a chronic disease of either Parkinson's or MS. I was about to get a needle in my back. I had a non trained or uncertified medical office receptionist assisting the doctor with an evasive procedure on her first day of work! Of course the doctor couldn't get the needle in my back, I was nervous.

It was a very painful procedure and as I lay shaking uncontrollably on the medical table, I was thinking that God sent me to this doctor as yet another test of faith. Yup, another test. I should mention that a week later I had the same procedure performed in the hospital and I never felt a thing. Professionalism makes all the difference! Get the right doctors to treat you. I had doctors and medical staff to explain things and calm me down.

God reared His head and showed me some compassion.

****

A Second Medical Opinion

I eventually sought a second opinion for my PD diagnosis and drove five hours every week to Temple, Texas to the Scott and White University Medical College. The year was 2003, and only months after I graduated. It's important to find the right medical doctors to help with your diagnosis. The problem with Parkinson's disease is that there is no test for it. Doctors run various tests to make sure you don't have something else and when all other diseases are ruled out, they experiment with specific Parkinson's meds to look for positive results. Basically, if the PD medication works, you have Parkinson's disease.

Reflection in my Mirror

I left the neurologist office in Temple Texas with the knowledge that I was a person with Parkinson's disease. The first thing I thought of, as I'm sure many of you have, was Michael J. Fox, and how he had been dealing with PD for the past two decades.

When I wanted to be a top National Bodybuilder I visualized myself standing on stage, the crowd roaring as I squeezed out the many muscular poses. *I succeeded.*

When I wanted to work in law enforcement, I imagined myself in uniform maintaining a crowd and calmly resolving a situation. *I succeeded.* I didn't want to become like Michael J. Fox, I mean he's a good guy but I did not want the same disease. *I don't want to succeed at that!*

Attentive to my walking, and now looking down at my feet, every step was focused – *heal toe* – *heal toe* as we returned to my hotel room. This had been my second visit to The Scott and White Medical College in Temple and my brother had driven across a few states to give me support and well, just to be a loving brother that he is. When we got back to the hotel we decided to freshen up before grabbing a bite to eat. We had our own rooms and as I stood outside of mine, I looked back at him and acted out by imitating one of the other patients we had noticed earlier in the waiting room.

"Hey, remember that guy that was trying to walk across the waiting room? *Varoom varoom*" I said as I mimicked the poor soul's stumbling attempt to move. We had a giggle as my brother assumed that I seemed to be taking all this in stride.

I stepped into the room and closed the door behind me. I was alone now for the first time to deal with my disease. I stood gazing at my reflection in the mirror. I thought about one of my favorite movies with actors Robin Williams and Robert De Niro, the 1990 movie "Awakenings". Not understanding my disease and not being able to distinguish the differences between Parkinson's and *encephalitis*, which was the disease De Niro's character had in the movie. I started to cry. The patients in this movie were given dopamine to revive them from their catatonic freeze state. That is the same medicine I will have to take. I cried more in the shower - no one could hear me there.

Evidently the PD medications were working as my diagnosis finalized. Medicine with levodopa relieves or diminishes some of my symptoms for short periods. There are other medications doctors can prescribe in the

beginning but that may depend on the stage of your PD

prognosis. I was placed on Carbidopa Levodopa right away.

I found out later that may have not been the right thing for

my doctor to do since Levodopa, over time, causes side

affects.

Here is a list of some possible side effects of this

medication:

- Abnormal thinking: holding false beliefs that cannot be changed by fact
- Agitation
- Anxiety
- Clenching or grinding of teeth
- Clumsiness or unsteadiness
- Confusion
- Difficulty swallowing
- Dizziness
- Excessive watering of mouth
- False sense of well being
- Feeling faint

- General feeling of discomfort or illness

- Hallucinations (seeing, hearing, or feeling things that are not there)

- Hand tremor, increased

- Nausea or vomiting

- Numbness

- Unusual and uncontrolled movements of the body, including the face, tongue, arms, hands, head, and upper body

- Unusual tiredness or weakness

Ref: http://www.mayoclinic.com/health/drug-information/DR600837/DSECTION=side-effects

Okay, *now* I know why I quit my job without notice!

I got what I wasn't looking for, a Bachelor degree, student loans, and Parkinson's disease. God is great, what a jokester!

****

Impulse Control Disorder - "Yeah I Quit!"

The year was now 2006 - my life is not the same. I'm not the same person I used to be, and my world has completely changed. I had been dealing with Parkinson's for three years by this time. I felt as though I was caught in a tornado's twirling wind or…am I swirling in shitty water being flushed down a toilet? I was gasping for air, suffocating, and confused. At work I had trouble concentrating. An officer in law enforcement must be able to handle stress. I would start shaking when stress hit. I couldn't let anyone see this because it would look like I was scared. I told the Sherriff I was thinking of giving up my deputy status and my side arm.

In retrospect as I look back at this whole experience, I may have wanted out of the sheriff's office and law enforcement because I tried an alternative medicine for PD. My wife had brought home a marijuana joint one day. I was shocked, to say the least, since I was a commissioned law enforcement officer. When you have a disease, and especially one like PD or Multiple Sclerosis, you may discover many professionals utilizing this drug for therapy. There are thirteen states that have now approved marijuana for medicinal use. I had smoked marijuana in my earlier years but grew out of that stage like most baby boomers. I felt I was a better cop because of that experience.

When I was in the Navy in the early seventies, I read a book about a New York City police officer named Frank Serpico. He-was an honest cop going against New York police corruption. The actor, Al Pacino played Serpico in the movie. My interest in becoming a law enforcement officer stems before that when I lived in Milwaukee. I wanted to become a police officer aid, however, Milwaukee had 5' 8" height requirements back then and I was only 5' 6". Instead I joined the Navy and didn't get into law enforcement until many years later. But I *would* be an officer that went by the book. I followed policies and procedures. And now I was about to do something that was against everything I ever believed in. I would commit behavior that was against my nature. A cop on the take or an over zealous power mongrel cop are not any different than a cop using drugs - in my book.

God forgive me!

I tried marijuana while still a commission master peace officer in Texas and it went against every fiber in my body. Talk about guilt! I felt as though I was betraying my fellow peace officers who put their life on the line everyday to stop people like me. Yeah now, here I was getting a hold of these drugs. Confidentiality will be important here and it this is why I do not mention one of my doctors treating me in Midland - not that he did anything wrong, but I disclosed this information to him. He, of course, was concerned due to the conflicting and precarious situation I was placing myself in. I explained to him how well the drug seemed to relax my right side. I felt that my right side, the affected PD side was normal after smoking. I asked him if he knew of any other patients that disclosed their marijuana use to him and his response was, "The only thing I can say is, of the others who tried using marijuana, all have claimed it benefited them."

Nevertheless, my medical use of marijuana went against everything I had worked so hard for. Imagine how I would feel if I would have gotten caught. Picture the disgrace, not only to me but, to my peers and the Sheriff's Office. I imagined the headlines would read: *Midland Crime Prevention Officer of the Year, SWAT member and instructor - busted for marijuana use.* Most likely the news article would not mention anything about my Parkinson's disease or the marijuana medicinal benefits, especially in Texas; the Bible belt capital of the world. Well, if any of this gets back to the "Midland Reporter" I'm sure they would find it interesting!

Headlines: *God hater retired - Midland Deputy used marijuana while employed with sheriff's office.*

The actual use of the drug while employed as a deputy was only taken within the last six months I had worked there. Not that that would make a difference. I actually stopped using pot months before I quit my job. The guilt was too much to handle. Because I did not want to get caught, I had figured- if I am going to take this drug for medicinal use, I should get a large amount at a time. I had a friend who was previously awarded "Teacher of the Year". This friend made a trip to Mexico for me. They were going to Mexico anyway and I had mentioned that there was something I needed. All I ever spent was $200.00 but I am still uneasy about this whole scenario, and still have nightmares over it. However, in real life, when faced with impossible situations, people tend to do whatever they need to, no matter the risks or consequences. It's not my intention to make this book a building block for the legalization of marijuana for its medicinal use, but the *right* to access it for medicinal use would have eased my guilt.

Eventually, everything went to pot. No pun intended. I actually stopped using marijuana (only because of my guilt) and moved on. Then the shit hit the fan! My wife came back from a registered nurse conference (there was no conference) and told me she was in love with someone else. Now I really needed out -out of the marriage, out of Midland, out of my house, out of my job. I wanted to run and not look back.

I wanted to end it all!

I know these things happen in many relationships but dealing with Parkinson's at the same time did was not helping me. I was thinking anyway that my marriage failure must be due to the disease. You could have divinely intervened here anytime God! But, you didn't.

After the divorce my son and I tried to make the adjustment. It was rough, both of us dealing with a loss of a wife and mother and me dealing with my PD. I should note he was dealing with my PD too. There are support groups for caregivers. It's important for readers to know this. Now I needed out of the house - it represented something my ex and I had worked hard for. I felt a desire to leave my career and move out of the state. I continually underwent a whirl-wind of emotions as I combated PD while trying to find the right sequence of medications to take. It took its toll on the two of us. On one particular day I suddenly quit my career law enforcement job without even giving notice. Shock over what I had done left me even more mystified. I had problems with sleep, mood swings, and everything. Maybe I was Bi-polar or maybe I just needed a change. It was probably from the guilt. I wasn't a real cop anymore, I cheated! My poor son – he held on as long as possible.

Serpico would hate me.

*****

A Mayo Clinic report states that certain drugs used to treat Parkinson's disease can cause patients to become compulsive. The drugs called dopamine agonists have also been found to boost patient's appetites for sex, food, and alcohol. Chemicals that help regulate movement and balance can also affect the brain's pleasure and reward centers. Dopamine is released in times of enjoyment and might serve to reinforce compulsive behavior such as gambling. It's one of the questions your doctor will ask you during a visit.

My compulsion started with lottery scratch off tickets. Previously (before PD) a year could go by and maybe I would purchase one ticket. Now I was taking lunch breaks from work just to go buy a ticket. Then a trip with my brother and father was planned to go to Las Vegas. It may have been my idea. I took three thousand dollars with me. Before the first night was over I lost it all. *Easy come easy go.* I took more money from the ATM. Then even more. I had to call the bank because I wanted more and they had a limit. It wouldn't matter if I won or lost. I just wanted to play, to gamble. I hated the way I felt. I could not wait to get out of there. I'm never going back for fear I could not control myself. This behavior was out of character for me.

What's wrong with you Dad?

With my son's mother in a different state, I now became the disciplinary parent, a job I previously let my wife perform. My son and I started having issues that resulted in his decision to live with his mother. He was not used to me handing out responsibilities or consequences. Not that I had to often; he is an excellent young man. I'm sure my mood swings kept him wondering what the hell was going on.

One day I walked into work and began my everyday duties. I only worked a few minutes when I suddenly decided to quit. No two week notice - I just quit. Guilt I guess, maybe PD impulse problems.

After my resignation from the sheriff's office I found a new position in my community at a local drug lab testing company. After being hired, I ended up changing my mind about this new job and quit the first day of employment. I never even showed up to work.

"What's wrong with you dad?" my son asked.

With my indecisive behavior, among other things, I understood my son's decision to move out. I didn't want to live with me either. I couldn't believe how much my life had changed in just a short period of time. My boy eventually moved to another state to live with his mother - leaving me in the "alone" star state of Texas.

I was a fish out of water trying to catch my breath, flopping from side to side not knowing which side to die on. I floundered as I suffocated; trying to breathe, mouth opening, closing, gasping. It's called Impulse Control Disorder (ICD) a known disorder among Parkinson's patients. I had it. I had decided to move to Wisconsin but changed my mind and searched for work in New Mexico. I interviewed for positions there and then abruptly decided to remain in Texas. Then I changed my mind again and decided to move to Milwaukee. My sixteen year old son was thinking clearer than I was. He had told me to go back to Milwaukee, that my family needed me. He saved me. I eventually vacated my house in Texas but was compelled to get out fast. I packed a few things and left all my possessions.

God you can have it!

****

Employment - Disclosing Health Issues

I moved back to Wisconsin where my adult children from a previous marriage lived. A friend took my possessions, and my house in Texas was sold just to get rid of it. I had lived in that home for 11 years. After moving to Milwaukee, I stayed with my daughter until I could adjust from the move. My treatment for Parkinson stopped but I could still get prescribed medicine. I felt as though I had lost my identity. I was no longer a husband, a home owner, a cop. I'm just an old man with Parkinson's disease. I immediately started looking for work but I was concerned as to whether to mention my disease during the employment process. I was uninsured and it became very expensive to continue my medications. Something a PD patient cannot go without! I researched medication charity sites that help people in my situation. I found one that helped with my main medication until I was insured. My professional work experience as a supervisor in Corrections and Law Enforcement sounded good, but who was going to hire me since I quit without notice? It wouldn't matter that I had seventeen years in law enforcement positions. Questionable behavior and work ethics is a concern for any employer.

Why didn't you stop me God?

Three months after moving to Milwaukee I found employment as a supervisor at Patrick Cudahy, a large sausage making plant. My B.S. degree was in Organizational Management and I believe my degree is what landed me this job. Great! I finally get to really use my degree. Maybe it wasn't a waist of time after all. Maybe I will bounce back and start a new life. Patrick Cudahy operated its own medical department in the plant and I had to decide whether or not to mention my disease. They could not do anything anyway due to the American Disability Act and discrimination laws. I had decided not to say anything about my disease, but during the examination I had to disclose my medication. Doctors know that if someone is taking Levodopa that they must have Parkinson's. He even asked the "question" and I reluctantly answered yes.

The plant was huge and I had trouble walking the distance. Plus after a few days, other supervisors had informed me that many of them work 60 plus hours per week and I knew with my PD related symptoms, I would not be able to handle the long hours. Looking back on that whole experience I sometimes wonder if they walked me around on purpose to see what I was capable of, knowing that I had PD. Others would comment, "What happened to your leg, you're limping? You weren't limping earlier!"

When the medication wears off (off periods) then my rigidity would come back. Three days later I called in and resigned. I sent them a letter apologizing for inconveniencing them and their time for the enduring employment process. It sucked. I was so happy to get that position.

Let's see if I can walk God. Nope! Sorry to disappoint you!

Patrick Cudahy didn't workout - now what? Ultimately, out of my sheer need for income and survival, I attained employment at K-Mart. Not to diminish the type of employees at K-Mart, but I had been in line for an administrative position at the sheriff's office. That's why I had worked so hard to get my college degree. And now, I was feeling as though I was working backwards. Will I soon be a greeter at Wal-Mart? Be nice to them - they might be one of us (PD'ers).

I only lasted seven months at K-Mart. I began having too many PD related problems. I was having trouble walking, thinking and concentrating. The rigidity was terrible. I had worked in loss prevention at K-Mart and that requires one to walk the store looking for thieves. When I started observing possible theft concealment from a customer, the stress caused me to shake. Well *this* wasn't working. I resigned about seven months later, but not until I had caught the assistant manager of the store loading his own vehicle with merchandise. Go figure!

I didn't give notice at that job either. I called in and explained that my PD symptoms interfered with my ability to perform the tasks. Another apology.

I continued searching for employment where I wouldn't have to walk around as much and got an interview at a county probation court facility in Waukesha. During the interview I explained and disclosed to them that I had Parkinson's but that I was capable to perform tasks (I hoped). I was honest in my explanation as to why I quit my career position in Texas. I honestly can't say that NOT getting hired had to do with Parkinson's or any ADA discrimination but during the interview I was asked how I felt about working with younger adults. Now *that* was a discriminating question!

I eventually filed for unemployment due to my medical condition, and thankfully, my claim was approved. I also filed for social security disability, knowledgeable of the nightmares of that process. You can read the cases on how hard the application process is to get approved for disability. With Parkinson's and having had over 40 years of social security deductions taken from my income, I hoped the process would go smoothly. When you file for Social Security Disability, you find that having the Parkinson's is listed among other diseases that permit you to skip a large part of the application. Parkinson's is listed under the category of impairments known as neurological. But the disability must be severe enough to significantly limit one's ability to perform some basic work activities needed to do most jobs. I was approved in only three months and received my first SSD payment by the sixth month from my application date.

Heal the disabled, God!

****

The Right Stuff

My financial situation was finally looking better-since quitting the Sheriff's Office but it had taken a few years. Along with everyone else in this economy, I could not find work as I am limited at what I can now do. I collected unemployment while searching, but then soon after decided to file for SSD. With SSD approval and payments on the way, I would also get a pension from Texas but I had to wait for the pension accrual date from the Sheriff's Office. That finally arrived and, while it supplements my SSD but it does affect the amount I get from SSD. When you put into social security for over 30 years, SSD is not reduced from pensions. I put in over 40 years. With SSD and pension, I would still be considered at the poverty level.

Symptoms change and progress over time and my emotions were bouncing around like a room full of super rubber balls. Hell, I needed to be put in a rubber room! God forbid that someone cuts me off while I'm driving; they don't want to see my road rage.

Could I be bipolar?

I was literally scared of blowing up and had to make sure I talked to a doctor about that. I didn't have insurance and could not afford PD medication. I believe the worse thing that can happen to someone with Parkinson's disease is to *not* have medication. And now, I had gotten myself in this very situation. Here I was a Vietnam Era veteran and spent four years on active duty in the Navy in war time. It had never dawned on me that I could get treatment from the Veteran's Administration. A friend suggested this to me and I was accepted after applying for health benefits.

The medical staff at the VA was superb. They asked all the right questions. They immediately began treating me for depression, bipolar disorder and Parkinson's. All my medical records were transferred from Texas to Milwaukee and I finally began the process of getting better. Well, we know PD is progressive and does not *get better,* but treatment - the right treatment- means everything. For any veterans out there that read this, the doctor that sees me for PD is a leading Neurologist from the Wisconsin Medical College. Many specialists are on contract with the VA, so you will get excellent care. There is no reason for me to disclose and list the medications I have taken because, like this disease, it will be different for everyone as we all respond differently to them.

I finally reached the point where I was not only getting better, but feeling much better too, although I still have my ups and downs. It took me about eight years to get to this point though.

I guess God is taking care of me - but on his time, not mine.

****

The Fear

When someone tells you have Parkinson's disease (a chronic disease) one thinks of the worst case scenario. That is because of the response we get from our peers. They usually respond, "Oh I'm so sorry to hear that." With that kind of response it would scare the hell out of anyone. That's why we need to do our own research. Based upon the probability that I did have Parkinson's, I began researching everything. To my great relief, I found out that I would not die from PD unless I choked from not being able to swallow. Some people with PD do have trouble swallowing. It's a question that doctors will ask you during every examination. I purchased a number of books, including "Parkinson's for Dummmmies." I know, its spelled "dummies" but you see, the letter "m" is on the right side of my keyboard and, my medicine is wearing off - my right hand is getting rigid. When this happens my fingers don't release properly from the keyboard. It's called freezing. I'll break from my writing to fetch some meds. It will take about thirty minutes for the medication to get past the blood brain barriers in my brain and begin providing dopamine.

Thank God for medicine.

I'm back, feeling much better too. When I'm in an "off period", which is when my medication wears off, a number of things happen. My right hand gets rigid. I lose my dexterity in that hand. My whole right side tends to stiffen. For some reason my family says they see my right shoulder raised up. I lose my gait when I walk. My right arm does not swing and I tend to plant my foot down flat rather then from heal to toe. The best way to explain this feeling is that you have to imagine flexing or tensing up an extremity. Do it, see how that feels? Imagine having that feeling all the time. That's how my right side feels most of the time. I have gone for walks when I was in an off period but where I had taken medication and I was waiting for it to start working. Many times I felt an immediate electrical current shoot down my leg the second the medicine started working. In stride my foot would go from flat footed to heal toe. That's how incredible the medicine works for me.

During doctor visits the doctor may ask you if you have trouble turning in bed. I have noticed a progression of turning problems. You're not on medication for PD while you're sleeping (at least I'm not) and when I try to roll over, my left side (my good side) has to do all the work. You eventually learn how to move (shifting movements) using one side of your body. The fear I have is that if my PD progresses to the other side in the future, I'll have to wake someone up by yelling, "Rollover please." I guess during the day I'll be yelling, "Hello, anyone out there? Somebody, wipe please!"

Oh God!

During the onset of my Parkinson's I was having trouble sleeping. I really believe that with the lack of dopamine one gets tired. They are now saying that sleep disorders can precede Parkinson's disease by decades. I found I had to take naps and they really helped. Just laying down and resting for ten minutes did wonders. I think that this also happens from the drastic on – off periods from medication. Dopamine agonists are sometimes used as an alternative treatment for PD. These meds can cause various reactions too. I was on Mirapex for sometime but that drug was known to cause compulsive behavior. Remember the gambling? The thing about Levodopa (the main effective PD medicine) is that with time, one has to increase the dose as your body tends to plateau from the dose taken. So here is the fear. This medicine has some serious side affects when one reaches high dosage or when one has taken Levodopa for many years.

There are many PD side affects, from what I'm understanding, such as: dopa resistant motor symptoms (postural abnormalities, episodes of freezing, speech impairment), and dopa resistant non-motor signs (autonomic dysfunction, mood and cognitive impairment, etc), and not forgetting to mention the drug related side effects such as: psychosis, motor fluctuations, and dyskinesias (diminished voluntary movements and the presence of involuntary movements, similar to tics). Motor complications also include dystonia (muscle contractions cause twisting and repetitive movements or abnormal postures). PD can be very disabling and difficult to treat. The important thing to understand here is that we, the patients, must research all medication and diseases that they (the doctors) prescribe or provide, and even their diagnoses.

We also must tell the doctor *everything* that is going on with us. Write it down and make a list before every visit.

Here is an example of questions or concerns I discussed from my last visit:

- I am having vivid dreams.

- I wake up at night with pain in my Achilles tendon which is caused from me pointing my right foot while sleeping.

- My on and off periods are too hard.

- My on periods do not last as long as they used to.

Past visits included topics ~~as~~ of insomnia, depression, mood swings, sexual dysfunction, waking at night with tears in my eyes, suicidal thoughts, compulsive gambling, stiffness, muscle aches, pulled muscles, torn tendons, dexterity dysfunction, blurred vision, etc...

I'm ready God, what else you got? Throw some more at me!

****

Support Groups

I attended my first Parkinson's support group in Midland Texas. The first time I went by myself and the second time my wife went with me, which also turned out to be her last time. I found myself in a room full of mostly elderly people. I was fifty at the time and I was a young attendee in that group. I can't remember much about the first visit because I was focused on the variations of symptoms the group represented. Most support groups meet monthly and they suggested that we bring a friend or a spouse with us on the next visit.

As Parkinson's progresses we will find that we will require support by caregivers, and our friends and family will become important caregivers. These caregivers are so important that they too need their own support groups.

Even more fear takes hold.

I brought my spouse to the second visit. She is a registered nurse. She knows about this disease. But I believe that being surrounded by, and listening to the other PD'ers and their caregivers describe their concerns and stories, scared her off. The topic that day was turning in bed - how to help the patient and the contraptions that can be used.

There are many different types of support groups and this one was an open group for anyone with PD. What I needed or wanted was a group that had people more my age. I could benefit from a group with people with this disease that were still working. Unfortunately, I did not know this back then and found this support group too depressing. After I moved to Milwaukee, I found a good support group at the Froedtert Medical College of Wisconsin. Young On-Set Parkinson's Support Groups are for people usually 50 years of age or under. Although I only attended a handful of times, it was through these meetings that I found a good doctor. These support groups provide various professionals and speakers that offer an abundance of useful information and/or activities. I have not attended a support group in some time but I would be able to walk through the door of any support group at anytime and be accepted with open arms. They might even ask for a poem. Here's another one of mine;

Stuck Inside

Like a tight rope walker
Unbalanced and unsure
Each stride is conscious
Absolute as I endure

As a lake freezes over
Or a train steams at gate
Ice water flows slowly
The engine wines with weight

As water has its cycle
Ocean, cloud, and then rain
Thinking too starts a process
But chemical breaks the chain

Frozen inside my body
My mind sets a course
Ready is my will
But action has no source

A tree stands in a field
Waiting for its breeze
A chance to feel alive
Limbs set free from it's seize

I'm a backseat driver
A progressive hindered guide
Out of control at the wheel
It's me frightened and stuck inside.

An important benefit to mention when attending support groups is that when you do attend, you have a chance to receive information on new research. I had attended a local support group in the past and I was notified of the 2010 Southeastern Parkinson's Disease Conference and Young Onset Parkinson's Conference that was scheduled as a web cast. These seminars are very informative and present speakers from all over the world that are in the know of new science or clinical research. Topics vary but you will hear medical professionals discussing research on Deep Brain Stimulation (DBS), future cell and gene therapies, intimacy and sexuality therapies, exercise programs and benefits. If not through a web cast, many support groups have their own speakers come in from the local and surrounding community to discuss medical news concerning the quality of life for people with Parkinson's disease.

Trying to Understand God and my Anger

It is understandable and somewhat justified to hate God when we do not have all the answers. Who is really to blame? We *need* to attach a reason to an emotional state. Could God have prevented all this from happening? No one knows God's plan. In desperation we all call out to Him and pray for ourselves or others. In response to our not understanding why something happens to us we look for answers. At our lowest point, we collapse and blame.

The day I held the gun in my hand I was at my lowest point. I was very angry. Louis L'Amour wrote, "Anger is a killing thing: it kills the man who angers, for each rage leaves him less than he had been before - it takes something from him." I was mad that I had Parkinson's. I was angry that my wife left me for another man. I was upset over my son leaving. I was disappointed in my failure to handle this disease. The disease had taken something from me and it was eating me alive.

I had to take control of my anger. I had to quit blaming God. "The best years of your life are the ones in which you decide your problems are your own….You realize that you control your own destiny." Albert Ellis. It was time to take control.

****

Free Disability Report

As your Parkinson's progresses and I'm sorry to say but it will, you may find yourself in a situation where you begin having trouble with your personal finances as I did. In my situation after my divorce - and losing that extra income, and from being out of work due to my disease, my credit began to falter. I tried to keep up with creditors as we all do but like my disease, my credit rating also progressively got worse. After I sold my home and relocated to Milwaukee and struggled with a few jobs, I fell through the ice. The Federal Trade Commission grants permission to access one's credit report for free once a year. I never bothered. In Wisconsin, I had a judge grant Chapter 128 debt relief which permits me to make payments to all my creditors without harassment or incremental interest accumulation. I had been anticipating my Social Security disability (SSD) check to arrive as I had been previously approved. In my anticipation to get my debt repaired, I had to wait for SSD to deliver. Unfortunately the law states recipients must wait six months for their first check. I could not pay the required payments as I was without medical insurance and paying out of my savings for medicine and doctor visits. The money was running out — *snap* — *crackle* - It's a thin layer of ice we all march on as we balance our finances and credit while unaware of a lurking disease that will throw a weight on your shoulders, certainly cracking the ice under your feet.

****

Submission

Taking control of my life meant I would have to surrender to the fact that these are the cards I am playing with the rest my life, joker included. I was 55 years old when I left Texas and moved back to Milwaukee, my real home. My adult children accepted me with open arms. They had wanted me to come back home for many years but my career and marriage in Texas kept me away. There would be a new transition in my life, but first I had to stop the blaming, and only then could I become whole again. We do not know God's purpose and we can be certain that one event leads to another. Psychologist, Elisabeth Kubler-Ross wrote, "There are no mistakes, no coincidences. All events are blessings given to us to learn from."

What can I learn from the manner in which I handled the situations while dealing with this disease? What were the mistakes I made? Were my actions even mistakes? How can I turn this midlife event into a blessing? First I had to realize that my disease was controlling me. It was controlling every facet of my life. I had to find a way to take control of my Parkinson's and use the disease. I had to place blame on the disease for my behavior. It was not God's fault. And as far as my ex-wife, she would have committed infidelity whether I had this disease or not. In retrospect there were many times in my life I had thought about moving back to Milwaukee. I thought about how great it would be to get back home to be around my other children and grandchildren.

These events led me home.

My youngest son has moved to another state but he is now in college. He is happy and we see each other every chance we can. He has a girlfriend; he is in a band and he has a job taking care of mentally challenged adults. That makes me happy.

Was this your plan God?

Never give in to Parkinson's disease but rather learn how to manage your symptoms.

This disease will not define me.

I began mental therapy and treatment with excellent results. Physical activity and exercise is also important and I began walking and even joined a gym. I already understood the importance of exercise as I once not only owned a gym; I had been a national bodybuilding champion. I know exercise will help keep my bones strong and decrease the loss of muscle tissue as I get older. Research has resulted in positive benefits for people with Parkinson's and people with PD have proven that spinning on an exercise bike helps reduce the symptoms throughout the day. I can attest to this fact.

Parkinson's disease is a disease about motor symptoms; however, mental anxiety and one's family are also affected. Everything must be addressed to move forward. Caregivers will be everyone that is involved in your life and they must be educated to understand the disease. There are support groups for caregivers as is needed. Stress factors that are elevated due to family situations or financial problems, or even your ongoing health care, may aggravate your Parkinson's symptoms. When you and your caregivers are treated through education and or therapy, you will no longer be defined by this disease. I no longer view myself as a patient, but rather as a person with Parkinson's.

Like most of us we do not want to spend our life alone. I wanted to fall in love again and find a partner. Not a caregiver! At an older age I was not going to go to the bars to find that person so I used a website dating service. After I met someone I disclosed that I had Parkinson's disease. It was important that anyone I would be in a relationship with must understand or learn about Parkinson's as they will be affected too as a partner. Fortunately for me the woman I met is familiar with Parkinson's as her mother has the disease too. We fell in love and two years later we were married. Life can go on as a person with PD but it would be most likely unsuccessful if I continually looked at myself as a *patient*. We are the same people we were before we were diagnosed.

My life moves forward.

****

Acceptance and Moving Forward

Living in Milwaukee now I spend time with my older children and enjoy grandparenthood like never before. A blessing in itself! Love will find you again if you permit it to as it has done for me. I am now married to a mother of two young boys 19 and 16 years in age. She is a teacher. Was it God's plan too for this single mother raising two children for the last fifteen years to find a good man?

My own parents had been living in Arizona and wanted to move back to Wisconsin so that my sister and I could help my mother take care of our elderly father. They live in Wisconsin now and are taken care of – and happy.

Was this yet another plan of God's?

****

Thanking Caregivers

Everyone that knows you and has learned of your illness becomes a caregiver. These people are; family, friends, co-workers, medical personnel, and disease cohorts who become your personal support group. We need to stay connected with all these caregivers. They will help guide us, listen to us, and assist us. They are there to give and receive, to share and to educate. Each caregiver is task oriented in that some are there to elevate our emotions, discuss our losses, and medicate our depression or disease or simply to remain at our side during our grief.

It's your job to help educate them about your disease. Within each caregiver you will find specific qualities. If they take notice and surround you, they have compassion. They want to communicate and be educated. They want to love and be loved. And yes at times, some caregivers need caring for too. You may be helping each other.

"There will come a time when you believe everything is finished. That will be the beginning."

~ Louis L'Amour

The above Louis L' Amour quote is what shook my soul when my son Dillon influenced me to move back home to Milwaukee. He was one of my family caregivers who *unselfishly* sent me away knowing what would be best for me. Also there for me is my sister, Sharon whose never failing love for God, strong family values and always wanting all of us together, was my *listener*. My co-worker and the best friend anyone could have, Lori who had the guidance to bring me back to faith and God, and for her compassion to care, her devotional love and sacrificing release. Other family caregivers are my son Michael and daughter Heidi for opening their arms and home with love and support. And my grandchildren are caregivers who bring joy and laughter while I get to be an educator again. And finally, my new wife Carmen, who allows me to trust and love again while my step sons Joe and Tony, reluctantly laugh at my quirky jokes. All have become caregivers. Look around, we have many caregivers to be thankful for.

****

Perception

Parkinson's is a chronic and progressive debilitating disease that strikes at the affected person from all sides. It can be managed with good doctors and the right medications. You can take control of the disease and if God permits, you may even find a blessing and a new purpose in life. One of the most influencing stories I have ever heard was from Apple inventor, Steve Jobs, who made a remark about choices. He said, "If you live each day as if it was your last, someday you'll most certainly be right." Since then he said, he has looked himself in the mirror every morning and asked himself whether or not he would do the same thing that day if it were his last day alive, and if he answered 'NO" a few too many times, he would change what he was doing. Although the connotation here was about not doing a job if you're not happy, and for you to find one that you enjoy, it made sense to me.

> *I am only one,*
> *But still I am one.*
> *I cannot do everything,*
> *But still I can do something;*
> *And because I cannot do everything*
> *I will not refuse to do the something that I can do.*
> Edward Everett Hale

Understanding

I was not to blame for the illness, a chronic disease that would affect me for the rest of my life. God knows we will get mad at him and He forgives. It is through God's grace we see things in the right perspective and come to a heavenly understanding that we need one another. We can utilize what solidifies as a causal dramatic change in our lives and share that experience in hopes of helping others. An event brings about our new purpose in life. We analyze our old purpose and we work on a new one.

Before I was diagnosed a co-worker and friend of mine, a female deputy was diagnosed with cancer. She has now since passed on. What purpose did she have after her diagnosis? She fought a hard battle but unfortunately lost. Or did she? Whether she worked and volunteered on cancer drives, provided funds or supported others with her disease is not a concern. We each take what we learn from others differently. Her situation made me look at my own disease and become thankful I did not have cancer. This may sound hardening but I do think that is honest statement to consider. But what I really got out of her battle with cancer was her infinite faith in God. Even with cancer and knowing she did not have much time left, she lived each and everyday to the fullest, right until her last breath. She could not do much, but she did what she could. She taught me how to live each day to the fullest.

I had been looking in the mirror and seeing an old man with Parkinson's disease who had no hope. I did that every morning. But I realized that I do not want to die an unhappy person. I had to change my perception of a person with PD. I'm playing with a new deck of cards now and I am holding in my hand - the joker. Some of you may call it Parkinson's. I call it my trump card.

God, forgive me - thank you.